Living on the Edge.

A medical doctor's autobiographical essay.

RM Rotcod

ISBN: 978-0-9997392-5-9

Bosveld publishers:
2177 Port Talbot place, Coralville, Iowa – 52241, USA

Preface

This is an autobiographical essay written by the author in 2006. Initially it was written for Rotcod's his own pleasures and memories, and perhaps also for Rotcod's children's memories of their parent one day.

No matter or individual referred to, is fictional. No real person is correctly named, although some individuals described could highly likely recognize themselves if they read the text.

This physician has had an amazing adventure along the course of a medical life. Rotcod has worked in very different healthcare structures, varying healthcare systems, and in multiple continents and countries. Rotcod has lectured and demonstrated medical techniques in three continents, and knows extreme 3rd world conditions, as well as best first world medical working conditions.

Before any person criticize aspects related honestly within the story, the author requests they consider whether they have the necessary life experiences, diversity of medical experiences, and depth of medical training to be qualified enough to criticize.

Living on the edge

We spoke of how in his healthier days, he had loved to walk on the hills of his African farm at sunset, as the day's heat waned. The next day he was under cardiac-bypass for heart surgery. Things did not go well and at the end of a very long surgical battle he either needed an immediate heart transplant, or we had to switch off all life-support machines. We eventually stopped the bypass-machines and switched off all the signs-of-life monitors. There was no way his own heart would make it beating out of the operating room. We had no realistic means to support that heart any further, nor a means to replace it. In that era there were no other heart pump technologies, other than full cardio-pulmonary bypass under anesthesia. It was an eerie experience for me to switch off all life-support machines on a brain-intact patient. The briefness and fragility of life was suddenly very real and tangible. His brain would be dead within single minutes of us switching off all the life supporting machines. The surgeon just could not get his heart to beat again.

The surgeon had tried for hours. The 5-vessel coronary artery bypass surgery had pushed our patient's heart over the edge.

I thought about my anesthesia patient long that evening, after I wearily got home. He and I had conversed happily, barely 24 hours prior, on his impending anesthetic and heart surgery. He was gracious and at peace with the risks that we had discussed, and he wished more to tell me about the beauty of his sheep farm in the arid Karroo semi-desert. I lingered longer than usual on my pre-anesthetic visit with him, as I loved desert places. I tried to imagine his farm that stretched from hill to hill, and onto the next valley too. All the great one-god religions were founded in deserts. There must be a reason for that.

I love the silence in a windless desert. I once stayed with Bedouins in the Arabian desert. In the evening I walked a mile away from the tented camp-site. In the moon-light five miles away, I could see large rock mountains protruding up from the flat sand-plane. I heard nothing from the desert. The total desert silence let me hear the rush of blood in my ears, that were attuned to the racket in bustling cities. In Africa I would hear the calls of animals and birds that awaken at night. In the Arabian desert it was just a deafening silence, at least initially. I hear nothing from the desert. You have to experience deafening silence in order to understand the term. I found by my third night that my ears had adapted and I no longer heard the blood rush in my head. I could then completely feel the silence of a remote Arabian windless night. It is strange to say, that one feels the silence, more than you hear the silence. Without any haze in the sky and without a single light-source visible anywhere, it was incredible how bright the stars were, and how many stars could be seen. Few stars twinkled. They just all shone immaculately. I could almost feel they were speaking to me. I lay on my back on the sand to study the heavens better. Every instinct in my body felt there was truly a heaven after life. I also strongly felt there had to be a greater power and a mightier being than I could ever fully understand. I felt very tiny beneath the blanket of stars, yet I also felt very secure and comforted.

The morning after I had spoken to my patient about his sheep farm in the semi-desert, I started his anesthetic. As I was preparing to inject the sleep drugs, and while injecting the first drugs, I was speaking again to him about the farm, and fire-red desert sunsets, and taking of us walking along the hilltops together, maybe one day. My soft voice, and those thoughts and images formed that man's last human awareness as he went to sleep. Both my words and the drugs caressed him to sleep and unconsciousness for the surgery. I kept repeating the image to him that he loved, and his eyes closed and I asked him if he could see it all. I did hear one sleepy affirmation, and seconds later he did not respond at all. He was anesthetized.

I intentionally distract all my patients that I am about to anesthetize, from their anxious thoughts and any obsessive fears they might have in their hearts. I learned to do this this following some early career anesthesia observations. I have seen so many times how a patient when awakening after anesthesia, recognizes me, and then completes the sentence they had only gotten half-spoken, at the point when by when my injected anesthesia drugs had kicked into effect. This was the start of the anesthetic. With my growing experience and repeated observations, I finally grasped that the last thought a patient has before anesthesia, is also that patient's first thought upon awakening after anesthesia.

Thereafter, I always tried very hard to make my patient's last thoughts, as they fall asleep, be harmless and happy thoughts. I do this because I wish them to wake up, back into those very same last happy thoughts and pretty mind-pictures, securely saved in their heads during the anesthetic. It was an amazing discovery seeing how the patients' heads preserve those thoughts and images across many hours of anesthesia.

I have also had a number of patients in my career, awaken after surgery screaming, and not from pain. I later found out they had awoken into a dream re-living some traumatic life event that was clouding their minds just before being anesthetized. So, I always want anesthetic patients minds to be filled with happy thoughts that I control, as they fall asleep, for they awaken back into those identical thoughts. I definitely have some control of those points. Thinking of my, now dead, desert farmer patient, I felt a flood of tears welling up, realizing that taking a beautiful hilltop sunset walk on his semi-desert farm was the last thing he ever thought about in this life. We just never knew at the start of the surgical day, what the nature of the ending of that day would be.

We live on the edge of life every day of our lives. We could be on a surgical table, we could be in a car, or we could be walking up a hill. We live life in its greatest fashion when we are closest to the edge of life. That edge is frightening, and sad, but can be exciting and invigorating too. There are many persons who love to climb dangerous mountain cliffs, and ride fast motor cycles. For that short time, they are savoring the thrills of living life on the edge.

I have had many patients die under my care during anesthesia. The vast majority died because we could not reverse their inevitable progress down the road they had come upon, into the hospital Mostly I had barely greeted them as they were half obtunded and we rushed to operate, perhaps to stop the bleeding, or something. I certainly knew nothing of them personally. I never had time to ask personal interest questions with those emergencies, and to build a professional friendship and bond. Many emergency patients arrived unconscious, and nearly all were bleeding badly. They simply were labeled "the ruptured aorta of Tuesday afternoon" or the "polytrauma of Saturday night". They were not persons with names. It was simply a technical scientific exercise. An operating room death meant many administrative white forms had to be completed, before we could go home. We also just wanted to go home and to get into bed afterwards, and the forms slowed us down. Those deaths never affected me too much emotionally, as they were simple exercises in medicine. Some you win, some you lose. You do your very best always, regardless. My old sheep farmer who had died, was not like that at all to me. I had bonded with him as a person, with a character and a soul.

One learns to have professional empathy in medicine. Professional empathy is when you feel everything for a patient, and you give everything you have, during the contract period of service to them. However, when your service contract is over, you forget about them. You just cannot carry a past day's sentiments with you into a new day, or it else breaks you. As a physician anesthesiologist you live life on the edge one day at a time, every day. It is notable to me that some of the most caring and empathetic doctors I ever knew changed careers in mid-life from a patient-involved one, to an administrative paper work one. They had gotten burned out from ever staring at the edge. When things go suddenly and unexpectedly sour with a patient under anesthesia, they can be effectively dead and over the edge within minutes. We may however, still battle to bring them back from beyond the edge for another half hour or longer before officially declaring them unresuscitatable and dead. That can break a doctor's soul. Luckily saving the patient is nearly the rule, and failure is rare in a ten-year period. No anesthesiologist ever has a patient-death free career. Although we are usually not at fault and seldom even get blamed for such events, we all silently flagellate ourselves questioning whether we could have done more for the patient. Anesthesia is the single most critical specialty in medicine. Anesthesia is practiced at the cross roads of illness sometimes threatening death, and death itself. As anesthesiologists, we try to direct the traffic at this intersection to help the surgeon drive the patient into a safe lane. The edge between life and death is never far away.

Still thinking about doctors having empathy for their patients, and then also the uncaring doctors too, I note some things. I have observed that some of the most uncaring, perhaps bombastic, doctors, in any specialty field, were the ones who thrived in the job until their seventies. I wondered whether being a caring person in life, is to be a burdened person in life. The uncaring doctors seem to survive better. Those doctors who care a lot, feel too much, and do not survive well.

A favorite medical thing of mine to do, is the obstetric epidural. The edge of life has two sides. On the one side people fall off, and die. On the other side new persons touch their feet down for the first time. They are born into the world. The pregnant laboring mother is typically not ill, everyone is excited about the coming baby, and then you take away their labor pain. They thank you profusely when the labor pain melts away, as if you have done something magic and wonderful. In truth, you only did what you were trained to do routinely. Furthermore, you helped someone who wasn't even ill, yet you get a big thanks. Pregnancy is a not a disease.

Best of all for me, is sometimes when a single mother progresses to a cesarean section and she has no accompanying life-partner. Then, I can hold their hands during the surgery. I talk to them to distract them from the surgeon's scalpel scratching the skin, and tugging on their tummy, that they may feel at the surgery start. It is bad that they need a cesarean section, but is great you can let them hold your hand. They always clasp it tightly, as they are more frightened than the married mothers. It makes you feel wanted, which is a good feeling. You are living on the exciting edge.

My most favorite obstetric anesthetic event is to place the newly delivered baby and the mother cheek to cheek. It is beautiful to see the mother and child become peaceful. I can tell they know each other. Occasionally a mother wants to feed immediately, while the operation is still on the go. The first time I received that request, I had to think for a moment if it was OK. Well of course it is OK! Hold the baby upside down so he lies over the mom's shoulder and help the mom lift her nipple and position the baby to latch on. It encourages the development of the breast-milk later on, and also releases endogenous oxytocic hormone to contract the uterus as the surgeon's sutures it up. Someone needs to help support the baby, as the mother is in an odd position to do it herself. One or both of the mother's arms might not even be free to help hold the baby. The baby can't lie the other way, or the baby then pushes under the sheets, into the surgical field of the surgeon. The sight of a feeding mother, especially one doing it for the first moment in her life, is one of the wonders of life. Everything in the world seems to make sense in those moments.

Anesthesia is strange in that in one day, one can both greet a new member entering the world, and bid another person farewell as they die an inevitable death. It is the cycle of life, and living on the edge.

One of the mightiest frustrations for an anesthesiologist is the uncaring surgeon. We conquered the pain of surgery in 1842, with the world's first anesthetic. Before that great year, a leg amputation meant living the awake-horror of having a seeming fire-hot scalpel blade slice your tissues from skin to the depths of your bones, while four strong men held you down. After that slashing in half of flesh, skin and muscles, follows the scraping-grinding feel of a saw dividing your bones in half. You scream and wriggle, but the four strong men hold you firmly down. The discovery of anesthesia banished those living horrors forever. Anesthesia has been called the greatest discovery in medicine. Some would argue penicillin was the second greatest discovery.

In current times we also have the skills and techniques to abolish post-operative pain, as well. Pain can be treated in high degree with opiates, but there are very miserable side effects and serious dangers when using opiates. A nerve block however, can totally treat pain and avoid all the dangerous opiate side-effects and risks. A nerve block takes a number of minutes to perform, and it also allows for a very light general anesthetic to be given to accompany the block, if needed at all. The end-of-surgery wake-up time when a nerve block is used, is much faster than the wake-up time after full general anesthetic without a nerve block. The advantages of nerve blocks for post-surgical pain relief are extensive. Those benefits, far offset the minutes of extra time taken to do the nerve-block.

The uncaring surgeon however typically finds endless objections to the anesthesiologist performing the nerve block, with “we don’t have the time” as the foremost reason. That lost time from performing the block is regarded by the uncaring surgeon, as a cost against which no patient benefit can counter balance. Invariably the real issue is that that surgeon has a personal social date planned for after surgery, the value of which to the unfeeling surgeon, exceed the patient’s interests.

A common joke surgeon’s make when we discuss the medical problem of pain after surgery is; “I don’t understand the problem. I have never felt pain after surgery in 20-years of operating.”

A caring anesthesiologist with the ability to do a skillful anesthetic and do nerve blocks, can offer so many benefits to the patient. The anesthesiologist takes great delight in having his or her patient be clear-headed moments after awakening after surgery, and also state that they are totally pain free. It is a such source of frustration when a surgeon imposes restrictions on the pain management plans for the patient. The patient then awakens after the surgery with partially resolved pain, despite the large doses of opiates used. In addition, the patient then usually also vomits from the opiates. When you look at that patient, you are feeling sad and sometimes angry, knowing you can do a better anesthetic that that.

I recall having a seventeen-year girl patient, needing a hind-quarter amputation for a femur bone malignancy. Call her Annie. Annie was a great athlete and she told me how she was going to remain an athlete after her amputation, and how she would compete in the special Olympics in one-legged events for America one day. She was being brave and clearly, she was emotionally carrying her anxious mom and dad who were not dealing too well with the life-threatening illness and disfigurement facing their daughter. Annie was also pretty.

We planned special nerve blocks for the young lady for her post-surgical analgesia. We were going to do this before the general anesthetic and surgery. As we started the nerve blocks, the surgeon sent a messenger to us instructing us to stop as there was no time to perform the block. Yup, the surgeon had guests for a dinner meeting later that day, we subsequently heard. The surgeon did not want to waste the 10 to 30-minutes extra time that the nerve blocks would have taken, lest it delay him meeting his guests in the evening.

Once we had the general anesthetic started and the patient settled, I approached the surgeon who had now finally arrived in the operating room, to join his junior assistants, and I achieved catharsis of my feelings. I informed him I was ashamed to be doctor that day. He, in surprise, asked me why. I explained I had had a young girl under my care, hardly different from my own daughter, who was about to have her beauty demolished by the loss of her leg and hip. She was having her soul torn into, and she still had to face the possibility of a cancer-death despite surgery. The least I could have done, would have been to relieve her post-surgical pain maximally and I had been stopped from doing that. I was trembling and the surgeon said nothing. I walked away with tears in my eyes, and on my cheeks.

We did eventually perform the nerve blocks, but only after the surgery and the general anesthetic. We had to vacate to another area to do these nerve blocks. It was very difficult doing the nerve blocks. Firstly, the girl was in severe pain and struggled to lie still. It was also difficult because we had no distal leg muscles to twitch in response to our nerve stimulator to help us blindly find the nerves. The entire leg was in a bucket on its way to the incinerator. We skillfully probed for the nerves in the remaining upper buttock region, with a needle inserted blindly through the skin. That is a part of medicine that requires high knowledge levels of anatomy details, and is an art-form uniquely practiced by physician anesthesiologists. Those leg muscles that could have helped us, were removed in the amputation. This was an unusual situation and challenge for us. We exercised our special skills maximally. Using novel innovative approaches, and alternative techniques, we got the nerve blocks done. It took far more time, than had we done this before the surgery. Worse, we caused that girl a lot of unnecessary pain as we had to reposition her a few times after the surgery, for the different positions that we needed to inject the various nerve-blocks needed. It felt unnecessarily cruel to me. Once the nerve blocks worked, the young girl became somnolent from the now relative overdose of the interim opiates she had needed before the nerve blocks set up. She no longer had the pain to offset the sleep effects of the opiates. There really is no argument that medically the nerve blocks would have been best done before the surgery. I wondered if the surgeon was in time for his dinner and how he enjoyed the meal. My feelings amongst many, included frustration, despondency and disillusionment.

We maintained Annie's nerve-blocks with infusions for four days. Annie had smiles for us the next day. I often, years later, wonder whether she ever achieved her goal of becoming a national champion one-legged special athlete.

That surgeon, who was very senior within the institution and also the head of his department, sought me out the next day to talk to me. He simply said, *"I just want to tell you, I have thought a lot about your words"*. He said no more and turned away when I had nothing to say. Subsequent to that, this same surgeon pointedly requested all his cancer amputation patients and all other major orthopedic cases to receive nerve blocks, done before surgery.

He also often requested I personally manage his very biggest and most complex cases. He became a great supporter of nerve-block pain control, and I admired him as a good doctor. I will never forget his humility in telling me he had thought a lot about my words. True greatness, has humility as part of it. Mahatma Gandhi had many quotes on humility.

You may ask why did I choose anesthesiology as my career? Well, I started out as an African small-town rural family physician, far from any big city. It was in a coal mining community of twelve thousand citizens, and had a small hospital. I obtained two masters degrees in primary care medicine and I loved the patients and the work. I saw general practice as my calling and career. I envisioned doing that through to retirement. Unfortunately, I had practice partners who had personal failings with respect to alcohol, morality, criminality, psychopathy and professional competence. After 7-years I decided to leave the partnership and to study a medical specialty. I chose anesthesia because it offered a fast track in four years of training to graduate with high-level competence. Anesthesiologists graduate at a competence peak, while surgeons by comparison graduate still in need a few more years of experience before they reach their professional skills peak. It was purely a practical job-based decision. Also, I had already had some modest general practice experience of doing anesthesia, and thought I could do it.

My first six months as an anesthesiology trainee was sheer terror. I had had no idea of what specialist anesthesia involved from my prior limited experiences anesthetizing only relatively healthy patients for small surgeries. My newly apparent ignorance, was overwhelming and my fear of killing a patient never left my mind. I had a racing resting heart rate of 100 beats per minute, every working hour, for the first six months of my training. It was like I was hanging on the edge of life and death with each complex patient's life, while they underwent major surgery. However, by the end of four-years of training I became fully confident and competent, and graduated well. A joke we anesthesia trainees often quoted, is that anesthesia is the art of poisoning someone to the edge of life and death, holding them there for four-hours, and then bringing them back from the edge.

Looking back to my days in rural general practice, I recall a day when I had one sweating patient in my consulting rooms who was ashen grey, and had chest pain radiating to the left inner arm. I gave the nurse instructions and dashed out to the very nearby small-town hospital to deliver a baby. My nurse assistant, in the interim gave the man nitroglycerin under the tongue and did an ECG. As I delivered the placenta, I was called to the hospital emergency room for another new patient with a fractured femur protruding though his thigh. I ran there, initiated IV therapy, and called for a helicopter to take him to the big city for surgery. At that moment, I was called back to see the lady who had just had the baby, who now had postpartum bleeding. On top of that, I got a phone call that my appointment consultation patients were all grumpy, as I was an hour behind schedule at this point. The obstetric ward nurse added in that the new-born baby was showing respiratory distress signs, grunting with rib retractions. I remembered I still had not even seen the gentleman back at my consulting rooms who had chest pain radiating into his left arm.

Everything seemed overwhelming and every one needed immediate attention. Of all these patients, not one patient's condition was not life threatening. I looked out of the hospital window and I wished for a moment I could have lain on my back under a shady tree on the firm bed of Kikuyu grass in front of the African hospital. I would have studied the swallows flying about high in the sunny summer blue sky, and I would have been far from this edge of life and death. I had never before, nor ever since, had a single day on the job where my job had so pushed me to the limits of total failure and potentially the loss of so many lives, all in one day. That evening I staggered late into my home. My wife asked after how my work-day had been. I just said smiling "Great. Everyone is alive," and left out the details. My training and experience, together with a lot of determination had paid off. The next day would be a wonderful day, maybe on the edge again, or not.

One of the greatest things I love about anesthesia is that one only deals with one patient at a time, unlike rural general medical practice. Every time, as an anesthesiologist, when I am involved in a cardiac arrest case and am performing life-support, I remind myself its OK. I know what to do, and there is only one crisis at hand. One anesthesia crisis is hardly stressful compared to five small-town general practice crises at one time, on the edge. One joke about anesthesia practice is that it is a stiff profession: One is bored stiff for 99% of the time, and scared-stiff for 1% of the time. When one is in that scared-stiff phase, you are figuratively hanging onto a patient's one arm, with your one hand trying to help them not fall off the edge of life and to death. The exhilaration is that that one is trained how to do it, and for the overwhelmingly large number of times, you succeed.

Another great thing about anesthesia is that one can forget a patient you have signed off on, in the post-anesthetic care unit. Generally, you are not treating them again. I recall having sleepless nights in my rural general medical practice days, worrying about my hospitalized patients. My hospitalized patients on a day could be an appendicectomy patient I had just operated on myself, an aged gentleman whose pneumonia was not responding to the first chosen antibiotics, and an asthmatic child who was becoming exhausted. The patients would still all be my patients to worry about the next morning, and the day after that too. With anesthesia, after one signs-off on a routine patient in the post-anesthetic care unit, one is truly done with them. Typically, there are no more decisions and responsibilities. I sleep much better as an anesthesiologist and each new work day is an entirely a fresh day with new exciting challenges and new people as fresh patients that I have never ever met before.

There are drawbacks to anesthesia too. Once again, my past rural African general practice experience gives me alternate perspectives. I recall many rural general practice patients bringing me gifts of home-grown garden vegetables or fruit-produce. It seemed like, if things got too bad for anyone to pay us money anymore, we would survive on community charity regardless and keep treating everyone. Patients would also sometimes pay cash for appointments just to show me a happy thriving baby I had delivered. Folks wrote thank-you letters and gave cards expressing gratitude for me having done little more than my expected daily job. I kept them all in a folder. Within single years the folder become thick.

Anesthesia is more a thankless profession. My file of thank-you notes and cards from my patients, as an anesthesiologist, is very thin. That is, even after 25 years in anesthesia practice. Patients relate to their surgeon who fixes them up and see them face-to-face repeatedly and at length. Patients' awake contact with their anesthesiologist is very brief, and we are usually not perceived as having done anything good or anything curative. The surgery is the curative event. I miss the positive patient feed back I got in general practice.

Anesthesia only has side effects and complications. Folks generally divorce those anesthesia negatives from the benefits of the surgery. Anesthesia cures nothing. Its only purpose is to make surgery possible for the surgeon, and tolerable for the patient. There is thus a very unbalanced and poor cost-benefit ratio if one's perspective is wrong. The fact the modern surgery could not be done without the anesthetic is overlooked. The result is any anesthetic side-effect or complication of any magnitude is intolerable to all, and especially the surgeon. You are messing up "his" patient. Living daily in a climate where that attitude dominates can drive one to look at the edge, as an escape.

Living my later life in North America, it was much publicized that physicians in the new millennium, are one of the top worker-groups committing suicide. Within this high suicide group, anesthesiologists were usually the single highest sub-group committing suicide. Within my life-time, I have had a number of colleagues jump over the edge. They all took a self-administered anesthesia drug over-dose to kill themselves. I recall one was a cardiac anesthesiologist who had been one of my teachers. I suspect he could not deal any more with the stress his surgeons caused him. I observed as a trainee, that they did not respect him. Another anesthesiologist who chose to step over the edge, systematically stole enough of hospital anesthesia drugs that it was noted and addressed to our anesthesiologist group. We had no explanation for the missing boxes of drugs. A year later my one work colleague was found, lying dead besides all the empty missing boxes of that one particular drug. An added factor that had pushed him over the edge was that his personal debts had become unsustainable. The reason for his debts was that his beautiful trophy-wife simply spent more money than my friend could ever earn. My dead friend was one of the sweetest most gentle humans I ever knew. I have a half-dozen more, related doctor-suicide stories for another day.

I think we should start blaming surgeons for messing up our anesthetics. Let's turn the paradigm around.

"Hey Joe! How the hell could you get a septic knee in the knee arthroplasty patient we did together? Do you know what a good anesthetic I did, and now she has to stay an extra week in-hospital. This is damaging my anesthetic reputation. People are going to think my anesthetic caused the septic knee that you operated on".

Surgeons can be both the bane of, as well as the joy in, an anesthesiologist's life.

I once *had* an Indian surgeon called Talib. When an anesthesiologist "has" a surgeon that means he has a regular working relationship with that surgeon of some duration. This was during a wonderful phase when I worked in an African big-business city metropolis of 7-million people. We anesthesiologists were all independent-practitioners, and we contracted personally with each surgeon we worked with. So, all working relationships ended up being where we both liked each other, and were both free to seek to work with someone else. I had worked with Talib twice weekly for eight years. Talib did not appear dynamic nor big nor bold nor beautiful. He was of modest stature physically and made no impression when he walked into the room. His hands were however technically magnificent, and he had mastered the art of minimizing unnecessary surgical movements. Each movement did something or he did not move his hand. That also meant he was time efficient and operated very fast. His vascular grafts had patency rates amongst the best in the city, and things generally went very well with his and my patients. In short, he was a phenomenal surgeon in his quiet gentlemanly way. I so enjoyed studying him operate as I peered over the drapes, or hanging sheet between him at the lower end, and me at the head of the patient.

Above all, he always looked for me at the end of each day that we had worked together. He would seek me out when the patients were all settled and checked back into their wards or the intensive care unit (ICU). He simply wanted to thank me for anesthetizing our patients, for him that day. That little "Good job" message just made me feel great. I would have done the fire walk with him, at his Hindu festivals had he asked me to.

Surgeons totally make anesthesiologists feel great, or feel terrible. It is a very one-sided relationship however. It is a sort of very patriarchal marriage, with the surgeon being the patriarch. In a patriarchal family structure, the father can be very loving and respectful of the wife. However, he can equally be mean spirited and the wife just has to eat it up. In the modern western world, the wife is an equal partner in marriage, mostly earns her own salary and has a say in everything. Many individual surgeon-anesthesiologist relationships have yet to evolve to be at the equal partner stage. Anesthesiologist see themselves as clever as, as trained as, and as talented as half of all surgeons.

Regarding the other half, we are just better all round. Unfortunately, we often do not enjoy sufficient recognition or appreciation from surgeons.

I overheard one North American surgeon that I was working with regularly, had said one day to a colleague, that I was messing around with his patient, except the verb used was reproductive in nature. I took offense and declined to work with him again. The university anesthesia departmental daily work-schedulers, were informed of my request in writing. Years later, circumstances transpired that I was forced to work with him. The operating-room staff-schedulers had no-one else with the requisite skills to be assigned to that surgery, for that day. I felt moved to explain my past avoidance of him and elaborated I saw similarity between him and the distal alimentary orifice. He apologized for his past comment, and we had a functional working relationship thereafter. Both of us were weary of the other, but we were got the job done and were professionally cordial with each other. I felt on the edge. I feared he would very readily lay a frivolous formal complaint about me to my head of department. Perhaps, he was wary of me doing the same to him.

My general approach to life and to work is never cause troubles for anyone, nor to tolerated unnecessary trouble caused by others. When drinking beer with a buddy I might rephrase that statement using terminology more commiserate with beer language.

It is a rare event that an anesthesiologist exercises his or her right NOT to anesthetize a patient for a non-medical reason. A patient can choose their doctor within limits, and equally a doctor can choose their patient within limits. We are however, absolutely expected to help all persons with life-threatening emergency medical conditions, when there are no immediate alternative doctors. This is a subject of ongoing North American ethical debate, and corporate employers of doctors do not like the concept that any employee has any freedom of choice. Employers of doctors want them just to be faceless milk-cows producing milk, or to be always-silent workers under instruction on an assembly line extracting income from the harvest of patients.

I recall, once when I was self-employed and working with the best surgeons in the world, a cocky lawyer whose wife I was about to give an obstetric epidural block to, make a loud-mouthed joke. I did not think he was joking, despite he slightly making as if he was. He said laughingly, perhaps sarcastically, that if I messed up medically on his wife, his law-partners at work were saying how much money he could sue me for. That was a threat.

I paused with the Touhy epidural needle already 2-centimeters into his wife's back, and looked at him thinking. I then said, *"I don't want to risk that then. I worked too hard on my career and studied too many long nights to take such a risk. I need my career for my children"*. I pulled out the needle, pulled off my gloves, said he that he needed to get someone else to help him, and I walked out. He was speechless and paralyzed in his chair. I did pause long enough to give him the opportunity to respond. His wife delivered his baby an hour later without an epidural. I was later told by the nurses the father was quiet and contrite during the delivery, and that the mother was loud and angry with him.

On another day, another lawyer said to me as I was preparing to anesthetize his aged father for elective abdominal aorta surgery and place an IV (intravenous) cannula in his arm, that he would sue me if anything went wrong with his father. The son was unsmiling and seemingly very serious.

I looked at the son and other family members, and after some thought I said I was cancelling the surgery for the moment, until they could get another anesthesiologist. I said I guess they would likely sue me for an equivalent of ten million dollars all going bad, but I would only bill for an equivalent of one thousand dollars (at that time), all going well. The odds seemed badly against me as the father's predicted perioperative mortality was 5% for his frail condition. I said I did not think this was a good gamble for me. My heart was pounding as I walked away. I feared the consequences of my actions. Equally, I was indignant and would not be bullied. This was living with my career on the edge.

I immediately went to explain my decision to my surgeon, and he said he understood. The patient got operated two days later, under the anesthesia care of another anesthesiologist, who was a colleague of mine. Apparently, the son of the patient was very polite to the anesthesiologist and gave him a gift of a bottle of wine afterwards as a token of appreciation.

Patients can really surprise one with kindness. I was once asked to anesthetize a partial hepatectomy for a pediatric surgeon. When we say "anesthetize a partial hepatectomy", it is doctor abbreviated-talk really meaning anesthetize *a patient* undergoing the surgery of a partial excision of the liver, done by a surgeon. The doctor-talk language sounds dehumanizing, but doctor-talk is just for doctors needing to talk fast to each other. The patient was from a foreign African country far North of my own. The unwritten rule for uninsured foreign patients was for the anesthesiologist to submit their anesthetic invoices weeks ahead, and collect the money *before* doing anything. Collecting money before a medical procedure was actually against a national ethical medical law. However, the incidence of uncollected monies and bad-debt with uninsured foreign patients was so high that all doctors broke the law, and collected money beforehand in such cases. Mostly they would have a third person hold the money, like it was in a trust fund. Authorities chose to turn an understanding blind eye to that. At that time, I was young in practice and naïve and had missed the chance to collect my money before the day of surgery. All my anesthesiology colleagues laughed at me, saying I was going to get paid nothing. It is practically impossible to collect money owed from a person in a foreign country. It is simply lost money.

I did my best, and the anesthetic and surgery went well. I next day posted off my account to the father of the child in the foreign country. I had ethical discretion in billing in my then country, over a fee range of 100% of a coded fee guideline to 300% of that guideline number. I figured to lose money I may as well lose a decent sum, and I billed for the maximum. Being a complex case with many special modifiers it was a very large sum. In my mind, I wrote it off to experience and forgot about the money and did not even send payment reminders. I knew it was a certain bad debt before I even started the anesthetic, but I was focused in delivering perfect anesthesia-care regardless.

Six weeks later, the father sent me from his North African country, full payment and a delightful letter of thanks for helping save his son's life. A gift set of charming ethnic art items from his family tribe accompanied the letter and cheque. It was nice to be wrong, very nice to be thanked, and very very nice to be paid.

My final memory to relate, of the emotional life as an anesthesiologist living on the edge, is about Christine's husband. His name was Norman. Those are not real names. He was a policeman and the last patient of my working day. He was to have his leg varicose veins stripped. He was a big man, but not obese. He seemed perfectly healthy, except for he had a remarkably high mouth hard-palate that caught my eye, as I examined his airway. I decided this was a soft potential marker for malignant hyperthermia (MH) and I decided to give a him an MH safe anesthetic as it involved no special efforts.

Christine was a dynamic girl and had one child from a first husband, who had died being shot in the course of police duty. Christine was a police officer herself too. She subsequently met another policeman and married him and had another child with him. That second husband, was Norman my anesthetic patient.

All went well initially and Norman went to the ward for an overnight admission. Norman had been nauseas after surgery and I gave a repeat dose of a new second generation anti-serotonergic anti-emetic drug. I also gave him a new injectable NSAID pain killer.

He snored heavily and kept his three room-partner patients awake. At four in the morning he stopped snoring and his fellow patients were so surprised they called the nurses. Norman was in cardiac arrest. An effective resuscitation was carried out.

I arrived back at the hospital the next morning and was surprised to find Norman in intensive care on a ventilator. I was bewildered about the turn of events, but he was doing well. Despite having a tube in his throat, Norman and I communicated intelligently with sign language and he had little pain. The intensivist physician's plan was to wean him off the ventilator soon that same morning.

Norman however, deteriorated rapidly over the rest of the day and it was soon apparent he had total hepatic necrosis. His consciousness deteriorated and before everything was understood he had brain death from intracranial hypertension secondary to the total liver failure. The optimum time window for a theoretical saving craniotomy, with a decompressing skull flap removal was missed. It was just a freakish rare, unexpected, fast moving, and predictable series of events. He was brain dead. We ventilated him for another two days as we tried to comprehend all of this, and pray for some miracle curative action we still could take. If he had had a timeous pressure relieving craniotomy, at the time he still could open his eyes, to save his brain, he would still have needed an urgent liver transplant within 36 hours, as he had no functional liver tissue left. It was impossible to arrange that. Total liver necrosis is an unwinnable illness.

We finally worked out things, when analyzing events long retrospectively. Christine's husband was an undiagnosed obstructive sleep apnea sufferer of the non-obese type. Norman was also a habitual non-mouth breather, we found out. He was fine in the day when he was awake and talking. When he was asleep, he tried to breathe through his severely narrowed nasal passages. That caused him to snore and breathe inadequately. The subsequent history we got from his wife of his snoring and apnea attacks was very strong, but we had never picked it up beforehand. His cardiac arrest was based on severe hypoxia occurring during severe hypercarbia after deep snoring all night with repeated periods of stopping breathing, the apnea attacks. His total acute liver failure was based upon the hypoxic induced cardiac arrest occurring during a severe hyper-adrenergic state, secondary to the severe hypercarbia that had built up. We did consider a Reye syndrome from the NSAID, but rejected that after much literature research. I also considered the new anti-serotonergic anti-emetic was the straw on the camel's back, and researched a lot of scientific articles. I later found potential explanations how it could have diminished the tone of the oropharyngeal skeletal muscles that pull the tongue and mandible forward. I have spent much time researching evidence on this, but it could not be proven. He did not have volatile induced hepatitis as he had had a volatile free anesthetic (MH safe anesthetic) and was never febrile.

Poor Christine was now widowed twice before the age of thirty, and had two children with different deceased fathers. The hospital owners agreed to pay an out-of court settlement due to one nursing record having been falsified. Vital signs recorded by the nurses for the evening had been recorded for two hours beyond the death and clearly had been filled out in the hours in advance of the crisis events. That implied neglectful nursing care. I don't think that changed any outcome though. Christine elected not to sue any doctor, as the hospital payment was large.

She was an attractive and highly intelligent girl, and I fully expected her to find yet another life partner easily. We remained in minor correspondence with each other for a few years.

By twist of fate, Christine's last late husband's father presented to me for anesthesia for a minor procedure six months later. As soon as I realized who he was and his family connection to a patient I had maybe killed, I was very rattled. This man and his accompanying family knew about me and were very positive towards me due to the concern I had always shown to Christine and the support I had given Christine. Examining the old man, he had the identical high palate and small nasal passage that his son Norman had had, who had died. Clearly this nasal anatomy was a hereditary feature. This man too was a likely undiagnosed obstructive sleep apnea sufferer. His wife gave strong testimony of the old man snoring a lot and having apnea attacks.

I declined to do the anesthetic, as I was still so emotionally burdened with Norman's death who had been only my second ever elective anesthesia associated death. My nerves were shattered. I wanted to step away from this edge. It was too close and vivid for me. I managed to impose upon a close colleague to do the case. I may have done the case, had I not found an available colleague willing to do it. The case required the administration of sedation for a gastroscopy.

My colleague had a very rough ride with the old man during the anesthetic. The case started as a gastroscopy performed under sedation-anesthesia. Due to Norman's father having recurrent airway loss, struggles to breathe, and his needing strong-handed support of his chin with an oral airway device to pull his tongue forward, my colleague was forced into a desperate plan. He decided halfway through the procedure, to intubate the old man's trachea and convert to full general anesthesia. The old man did go home alive, I am glad to tell. We strongly advised that he seek otorhinological advice about his nasal passages, with a strong view to operating his nose inner passages, to open them up more.

Subsequent to all of this, and my ongoing research, I have acquired expertise in obstructive airway disease and have lectured at national conferences on the subject. I have delved into the role of serotonin receptors in glossopharyngeal muscle tone and the effect of anti-emetic drugs upon that. I communicated with pioneer researchers in serotonin receptors in Russia and Switzerland. It seems the anti-serotonergic anti-emetic drug that we gave Normal was less selective for the good serotonin drug receptors on the cells, than the drug manufacturers led us to believe. So, the second dose of that anti-nausea drug after Norman's anesthetic, likely weakened the muscles that keep the facial airways open when he slept, by blocking in the brain some of the "bad" serotonin receptors on other brain cells, slightly as well. In addition, the situation was likely worsened by the fact that, maybe all obstructive sleep apnea suffers have a congenital susceptibility to that airway muscle weakening drug effect that normal persons do not have. I am working on writing this all for a case report in the scientific literature. Medical science is still very incomplete. Doctors would likely all be in shock, if medical science still to come, in the future one day, could explain how close to the edge we treat all patients every day in present times.

Christine's children were four and six years old when they lost Norman, their dad and adopted dad respectively. I was 6-years old and my brother 4-years old, when we lost our father in an African hunting accident. I grew up wondering about the man my father was. I thought of Christine and her two boys often. I mostly wonder if a different anesthetic, with different drugs would have left him alive. I don't blame myself for Norman's death, I just wonder about things a lot. That is life. The final book on medical science is not yet written. We just do the best we can as imperfect practitioners, treating imperfect patients, using imperfect science. By very large, we medical doctors do phenomenally well, but perfection in medicine has to remain the hard striven for goal.

Anesthesiologists, more than any other physician doctor, practice medicine on the very edge of life and death every day and with every case. Sometimes, in the course of a day's work, an old life makes place for a new life. When my wife and I were in a hospital elevator one night, riding sadly and silently to see my wife's mother on her deathbed before they wrapped her and removed her, a fellow man elevator passenger was smiling massively and babbling joyously to us, as total wide-eyed strangers. His son had just been born minutes earlier, and he was rushing to the canteen to get his exhausted wife a cup of coffee. It sounded to me as if when my mother-in-law gave up her spark of life, a new baby-to-be-born grabbed it and popped out of his mother to start crying. The spark of life got passed on. It is the cycle of life.

When one life crosses the edge having an untimely death, another life, somewhere, arrives at the edge to start a sunny earthly existence. On any working-day, an anesthesiologist can also be with each of those persons on the edge. The anesthesiologist can then be the last human, or the first human to ever hold and feel those patients' hands with his or her own bare hands, while the patient's hands are warm and pulsing.

I need to relax now. I am going to ride my Italian motorbike on a quiet winding country road, to get a mental break. I hope no deer suddenly crosses the road in front of my motorbike. There is never escape from living on the edge.

The end.

Other books by **RM Rotcod**:

- **Tedoop and the Best Foot Print in the Sand.** (short story - read in 90 minutes)
    - Tedoop is a philosophical beach crab who is technology wise. He sneaks into ladies' handbags on the beach, and swiftly types text messages on the smart phone, to his seagull friend in Australia. Tedoop is friends with all the creatures in the air and in the water along the coral reef. He inspires and motivates everyone around him. This is an uplifting book for any adult struggling with the harsh realities of life, due to them still having the pure heart of a child. It is equally a book for the pre-teen or young teenage child who is straining with childhood due to them already having the noble soul of an adult.

Find this book on **Amazon** as an eBook or a print book. Search under the author name of **RM Rotcod**.

Other books by **RM Rotcod**:

- **The Mars Doctor**. (full length 310-page novel)
    - NASA sends 14 astronauts to Mars on their first ever manned mission to Mars. It is scheduled as a 3-year round-trip. The story is told by the accompanying space-doctor. The mission is ill-planned, poorly engineered, politically rushed, and the crew includes some human misfits. It becomes a story of survival dealing with unthinkable medical catastrophes occurring in space where treatment resources are extremely limited. Space-ship disasters occur again and again, one on top of the other. The story is a contemporary science-drama of human struggles to survive impossible disasters. This inspiring story has an unpredictable ending. The very last written line will never be forgotten. Be chilled, be thrilled and be uplifted. Feel horror at the brutality of some crew, and then later be warmed by others showing incredible human tenderness in unexpected developments. The story is real and tangible.

Find this book on **Amazon** as an eBook or a print book. Search under the author name of **RM Rotcod**.

Other books by **RM Rotcod:**

- **The meaning of Depression: A trout fly-fisherman's perspective.**
  - Despite the dark title, the story is charming. It is autobiographical and is a simple sharing of thoughts relating to how trout fly fishing appreciation requires a certain psychological frame of mind. In converse, trout fly- fishing, if properly approached mentally, has positive effects back into the fisherman's soul. The author shares cute experiences that can be fascinating to the person ignorant about fly-fishing, or enchanting to the person who has already embraces fly-fishing as a sport of the soul.
  - This is a very short story of 2600 words.
  - It is presently available for free as a print copy only, from the publisher, one copy per person.
  - Mail $3US per copy, to Bosveld Publishers at 2177 Port Talbot place, Coralville, Iowa 52241, USA, to cover postage, within the USA.

It may also become available as part of a collection of short stories in a future eBook and printed form via Amazon, in about 2021.

Other <u>future</u> books by **RM Rotcod**:

- **A military Rifle's story:** This book is in the process of being written, and is about a world War one military rifle.
    - The rifle tells the story. It describes its experience from being manufactured, to participation in the horrors of trench warfare. The rifle has no sense of time as humans do, and gives detailed accounts of a bullet being fired and coming to rest eventually a half second later, as if the saga took place over ten minutes. Warfare is seen as graphically horrific, as never before portrayed. The rifle is a devoid-of-emotion story teller, making the described horrors even more graphic.
    - The story continues in the post-war era and meanders through hunting in rural Africa, and eventually its owner's suicide using the rifle. Possession of the rifle changes hands a few times, and its journey thereafter is unusual. A noble destiny is however serendipitously fulfilled.
    - The rifle's journey is completed when the rifle dies from rust due to a roof leak in an old farmhouse dripping down a wall onto which the rifle is mounted for display. As it rusts, for the first time the rifle can feel emotion and events occur

that bring the story to the happiest possible conclusion imaginable.

- There are very strong autobiographical elements of the author in the story, although the story is, however, presented only as fiction.

The title of the book is being withheld until publication. The publication date is targeted for the year late 2020 or early 2021. Follow the author **RM Rotcod** for its publication on Amazon. The author can also be followed in Google searches.

Other future books of **RM Rotcod**:

- **The girl who hears the trees talk**. This forthcoming book is about a peri-pubertal girl who suffers from visual and auditory hallucinations.
  - She has an exceptionally high intelligence and struggles to handle her coming of age, together with these strange visual images and sounds that she experiences. Her devoted father has the means to assist her in her pursuit of solving the mysteries she becomes aware of.
  - She visits very special trees in very special places around the world, and gathers the information clues about her hallucinations. Maybe the hallucinations are real images and voices, uniquely seen and heard by the girl.
  - Each tree in the story is a real tree the author has seen, photographed and touched somewhere around the world. Readers will be able to trace these real trees. A few selected trees in the story, that are real, are to be found in very exotic but reachable places around the world. Those specific trees actually have engraved metal plaques and some coins hidden in their bases, by the author. Clues to their discovery is concealed within the book and prizes are available it they are ever

returned to the author. The book will give more information within the story.

The publication title of the book, is being withheld until final publication. The publication date is targeted for the year 2021. Follow the author **RM Rotcod** for its publication on Amazon. The author can also be followed by Google searching.

Other future books by **RM Rotcod**:

- **A medieval story about a mentally twisted court jester and a Noble bachelor king**, in a fictious kingdom in the South of old France.
    - This story is currently in writing and targeted for completion by early 2022. The time setting coincides with the third Crusade to free the Holy land from its Muslim control under Saladin. The plot is an extreme saga simulating modern corporate type internal intrigue, current educational institutional type of internal rivalries, and corruption of human management systems. The setting is however set in medieval times. Anyone who had ever been subjected to anonymous false accusations in a modern work setting will completely feel the reality within this fictional story.
    - The description of having a Machiavellian plot within the story, will be an understatement. The worst of human conniving, scheming and betraying behavior is the norm for court behavior in this kingdom. A very unlikely character helps find decency and nobleness in people, and helps them find it in themselves. The true hero of the story will be a mystery right to the last page, and

then the reader will still wonder if they understand that character.

- A reader's conclusion will certainly be that although we have amazing technologies and phenomenal institutions and governance now in this new millennium, that human behavior is as primitive today as what it 500 years ago, and even thousands of years before that too.
- There is however encouragement for the reader and it is possible even a cynic will find upliftment and hope for life and mankind by the end of the book.

The publication title of the book, is being withheld until actual publication. The publication date is targeted for late 2021. Follow the author **RM Rotcod** for its publication on Amazon. The author can also be followed by Google searching.

Other future books, by **RM Rotcod**:

- **The losing rugby side**. This is a story about a school's one B-side age-group rugby team, made up of reject players and coached by a reject coach school-teacher.
    - It is a story of school boy losers who have to first learn how to lose, before they can learn how to win. This they do in Rugby. The coach has to discover hope for himself, faith in himself and improve his own self-image before he can guide the rugby team towards improvement.
    - The story's conclusion is in fact not the conclusion of the bigger story. The final chapter ends there, but the reader will grasp that the real story is much bigger and projects onwards. The real story starts at the end of the book, and will be unwritten. Most readers will identify themselves with a player or two, or recognize a player or two as someone they know.
    - The story touches on some of the greatest actual rugby games ever played. It will be hard for a reader to not conclude that rugby is maybe one of the ultimate sports in the world. A deeper and true understanding of what a team is, will be realized. Every person of every personality type

can find a unique role for themselves in teams of all forms, in real life.

The actual publication title of the book is being withheld until publication. The publication date is targeted for the year 2021. Follow the author **RM Rotcod** for its publication on Amazon. The author can also be followed by Google searching.

Other future books, by **RM Rotcod:**

- **The best buddy of Jesus Christ, the boy.** This book in the planning and draft writing phase, has involved much research into the history of the ancient Palestine regions, and even pre-history periods.
    - Rotcod has tramped the lands and waters of Bethlehem, Nazareth, the sea of Galilee and the river Jordan in all of Israel, the Westbank and Jordan. The novel in preparation will be respectful of all faiths and belief systems. The story, is definitively only a fantasy born in the author's head. It is not being presented as theological argument. Rotcod is inspired by the belief that all persons have potential to be good persons, including the wicked.
    - Two little boys grow up together in the hills herding sheep and learning carpentry. The buddy character is slightly an Asperger's syndrome child, but finds fascination in his incredibly clever and prematurely wise little friend who studies the ancient Hebrew bible and discusses theology with the Rabbis at Capernaum.
    - The friend is the story teller, and tells of his clever friend's life, his growing up and his life ending. He observes it all from the side of the crowds and the

followers of his best life-friend. The story-telling friend is largely a silent and reclusive person, but one who the inspiring and eloquent talkative friend chooses to connect with and embrace spiritually. There is a hidden purpose in that friendship.

- The book is a window into the life and times of the Palestinian region 2000-years ago. It will inspire all persons reading it, and motivate them to love their neighbors more. There will be clear psychological and personality parallels between original imperfect and bad characters of those biblical times, and similar persons we all meet in our present lives.

The actual publication title of the book is being withheld until publication. The publication date is targeted for the year late 2021 or early 2022. Follow the author **RM Rotcod** for its publication on Amazon. The author can also be followed in Google searches.

Made in the USA
Monee, IL
04 November 2026

67352875R00036